Eye Massager 101

Everything You Need to Know About This Amazing Device

Gregory H. Cayer

Copyright

Table of contents

Dedication

To all the people who suffer from eye strain, fatigue, and stress, this book is for you. I hope that by reading this book, you will learn how to use an eye massager to improve your eye health, relax your mind, and enhance your well-being. I also hope that this book will inspire you to take care of your eyes and appreciate the beauty of the world around you.

I dedicate this book to my family, friends, and mentors, who have supported me throughout my journey as a writer and an eye care enthusiast. Thank you for your encouragement, feedback, and love. You are the reason I write.

Lastly, I dedicate this book to you, dear reader, for choosing to invest in yourself and your eyes. I hope that this book will provide you with valuable information, practical tips, and helpful insights on how to use an eye massager effectively. I hope that this book will make a positive difference in your life.

About Author

Gregory H Cayer is an eye care enthusiast. He has been using an eye massager for over five years and has experienced its benefits first hand.

He decided to write this book to share his knowledge and passion for eye massagers with others who want to improve their eye health and well-being.

Gregory has a degree in journalism and has written for various publications, blogs, and websites. He enjoys researching and writing about topics related to health, wellness, and technology.

Introduction

Is it possible that you have ever experienced feelings of exhaustion, agitation, or irritation after spending a long day reading, working on tasks, or gazing at screens? Do you have trouble concentrating, when you try to go to sleep, or when you want to feel happy? You may be experiencing eye strain, dryness, or weariness if any of the following questions apply to you. These pervasive problems affect millions of people all around the globe, especially in this day and age of digital devices and an abundance of information.

However, you shouldn't be too concerned since there is a solution to alleviate the pressure on your eyes and improve the quality of your life. An eye massager is a piece of equipment that has the potential to provide your eyes with a massage that is both calming and reinvigorating. Providing your eyes with a pleasant and soothing experience that helps relieve strain, dryness, and fatigue is the purpose of an eye massager, which is a device that utilizes heat, vibration, and music to achieve this. Additionally, eye massagers have the potential to boost oxygen supply, blood circulation, and metabolism in your eyes, all of which may contribute to an overall improvement in your health, well-being, and vision.

All individuals who are interested in enhancing their lifestyle and taking better care of their eyes might benefit from the use of an Eye Massager. You may use an eye massager to quiet your eyes and clear your mind whether you're a worker, student, reader, gamer, or tourist. The Eye Massager is a terrific addition to your daily routine because it is affordable, lightweight, and easy to use.

But not every eye massager is created equally. You must pick an eye massager depending on your needs and interests from the various models, varieties, and functions that are accessible on the market. Additionally, you must grasp how to integrate an eye massager into your routine and employ it safely and productively. For this reason, we created this book specifically for you.

<u>**You will learn all there is to know about Eye Massager in this book, including:**</u>

- ★ **How to integrate an eye massager into your daily routine**
- ★ **How to use an eye massager safely and effectively**
- ★ **How to add extra tips and tricks to your eye massager experience**

By the time you complete reading this book, you will know how to employ an eye massager to help you sleep better and feel better overall. Additionally, you may enjoy the benefits of an eye massager with your spouse, family, or friends by sharing your experience with them.

Are you prepared to experience the exciting world of eye massagers now? **In that case, let's get moving!**

Chapter 1

Safe and Effective Use of Eye Massager

An eye massager works by gently massaging, heating, and vibrating the acupoints around your eyes to help you relax and see better. Additionally, it may play pleasant sounds and music to help you unwind. This chapter will show you how to use and set up your eye massager, how to pick the optimal mode, temperature, and length of time for your sessions, how to clean and maintain your eye massager, what the dos and don'ts while using it, and how to address frequent difficulties with it.

How should I build and use my eye massager?

You must take the following procedures to set up your Eye Massager device:

★ Use the provided USB wire to charge the Eye Massager device. When the device is charging, the charging indicator goes red, and when it is entirely charged, it turns green.

★ To activate your eye massager, hold down the power button for three seconds. Both the power indicator and the greeting sound will glow.

★ Adjust the elastic straps to tighten or relax the headband to meet the size of your head. Make sure the device fits securely around your eyes without being too tight or loose.

★ Use Bluetooth to attach your Eye Massager device to your smartphone. The Eye Massager app enables you to stream music or sounds from your phone and alter the device's settings. As an alternative, you may manually adjust the settings using the buttons on the device.

★ Press the device's or the app's start/pause button to begin an Eye Massager session. By the mode, temperature, and time you have selected, the device will start massaging your eyes. Pressing the same button twice will interrupt and resume the activity.

★ You may either wait for the Eye Massager session to complete automatically or cancel it by pushing and holding the start/pause button for three seconds. There will be a goodbye sound and the device will discontinue massaging your eyes. After five minutes of inactivity, the device will shut off and the power indicator will flicker.

How do you determine the optimal temperature, mode, and amount of time for your eye massager session?

There are five various modes, three temperature settings, and four duration selections accessible for your eye massager. Your eye massager session may be personalized to your preferences and tastes. The following tips will help you determine the appropriate mode, temperature, and amount of time for your eye massager session:

Mode

There are five modes available: **Custom, Energize, Refresh, Relax, and Sleep.** To match varied requirements and moods, each mode delivers a unique combination of pressure, heat, and vibration patterns. For instance, the Energize mode is supposed to improve alertness and productivity, while the Relax option is meant to help you relax and decrease stress. By picking the Custom mode and manually tweaking the vibration, heat, and pressure parameters, you may even create your mode.

Temperature

Low, medium, and high are the three accessible options. Your comfort level and the blood flow and metabolism in your eyes are both influenced by temperature. For instance, low temperatures are excellent for soothing and cooling your eyes, while high temperatures are good for invigorating and warming them. If you'd like, you may also deactivate the heating function.

Duration

Ten, fifteen, twenty, and thirty minutes are the possible durations. The duration of your Eye Massager session determines both its effectiveness and intensity as well as your availability of time. For instance, 10 minutes is adequate for a brief break and refreshment, while thirty minutes is plenty for lengthy rest and recovery. By picking the Custom option and manually altering the time frame, you may also set the duration.

How should your eye massager be maintained and cleaned?

The following steps are important to maintain the cleanliness and performance of your eye massager device:

★ To get rid of any dirt, sweat, or oil, wipe the device clean with a soft, dry cloth after each use. When cleaning the device, avoid using water, alcohol, or detergent as these materials may cause injury or irritate your skin.

★ Remove the headband from the device once a week and give it a brief wash in warm, soapy water. Before reattaching it to the device, give it a thorough cleaning and allow it to air dry fully. To retain the suppleness and quality of the headband, avoid washing or drying it with bleach, fabric softener, or dryer.

★ When not in use, store your eye massager in a cool, dry, and well-ventilated environment. To extend the device's lifespan and increase its function, keep it free of the direct sun, high heat, moisture, and dust.

★ To protect the battery on your eye massager from running out of power or dying, charge it often. Avoid overcharging the item or keeping it plugged in for a lengthy time as these acts could lead to overheating or fire hazards.

What should and shouldn't be done when employing an eye massager?

You must adhere to the following dos and don'ts to use your eye massager equipment correctly and effectively.

> *If you have any eye diseases, injuries, infections, or surgeries, or if you are expecting a child, breastfeeding a baby, or have any other medical implants such as a pacemaker, please check with your doctor before using an eye massager.*

> *Please only use the eye massager on your eyes; do not use it on your mouth, nose, ears, or neck.*

➤ *Please only use the eye massager for the prescribed time and purpose; do not use it more than twice a day or for more than 30 minutes per session.*

➤ *Before using the Eye Massager, please take out any jewelry, contact lenses, glasses, cosmetics, and other materials that can create interference with the device.*

➤ *When utilizing the eye massager, do not distract your focus from tasks like working, watching, or reading. Instead, concentrate on relaxing your eyes and thoughts.*

➤ *If you have any allergies, skin sensitivities, or bad reactions to the gadget or the material of the headband, do not use the Eye Massager.*

➤ *If the eye massager is not completely charged or if it is broken, damaged, or malfunctioning, do not use it. This also applies to the headband.*

➤ *Avoid using an eye massager if you are feeling unwell, lightheaded, or sleepy, or if you are affected by drugs, alcohol, or medication.*

➤ *Avoid using an eye massager while operating machinery, driving, or engaging in any other activity requiring attention or focus.*

> *Avoid using an eye massager in dangerous environments, such as those with strong magnetic fields or radio waves, water, fire, or electricity.*

How can I handle regular troubles with my eye massager?

You may try the following remedies if your Eye Massager gadget isn't operating properly.

Issue: There is no _method_ to turn on or off the device.

Remedy: Inspect the battery life and, if needed, charge the device. To turn the device on or off, press and hold the power button for three seconds. For

Issue: The device is unable to establish a Bluetooth connection with the smartphone.

Fix: Verify that both the device and your smartphone have the Bluetooth capability switched on. Ensure that the smartphone and the device are 10 meters away. Verify that no other Bluetooth devices are causing the connection to fail. Try again after restarting the device and the smartphone.

Issue: The eye massager isn't performing its job.

Fix: Ensure that the item fits securely and pleasantly over your eyes. Verify that the duration, temperature, and mode settings meet your needs and preferences. If required, adjust the settings manually or via the app. For support, get in contact with customer service if the situation persists.

Issue: The device emits weird scents or noises.

Remedy: Immediately halt using the device and unplug it from the power source. Examine the device for any damage, dust, or strange materials, as well as the headband. As advised, clean both the gadget and the headband. For support, get in contact with customer service if the situation persists.

Issue: The item irritates, hurts, or pains the skin.

Remedy: Immediately quit using the device and remove it from your sight. Look for any evidence of an allergy, wound, or infection on your skin and eyes. See your physician if required. Wait until the problem is repaired before using the device once more. For support, get in contact with customer service if the situation persists.

Chapter 2

Including An Eye Massager In Your Everyday Life

An eye massager is a gadget that applies gentle pressure to promote blood flow to the acupoints around your eyes, hence decreasing dryness, discomfort, and tiredness. It may help elevate your emotions, decrease wrinkles and dark bags under your eyes, and enhance your vision. This chapter will illustrate the different uses and times of day for which you may use an eye massager, as well as how to blend it with other eye care products or treatments for optimum outcomes. Additionally, you will learn how to operate an eye massager for a nice and peaceful experience with your loved ones, friends, or spouse.

How Should an Eye Massager Be Used in the AM, PM, and Evening?

If you have a long day ahead of you, utilizing an eye massager in the morning can help you wake up and rejuvenate your eyes. Ten to fifteen minutes before or after breakfast, or while preparing for work or school, is when you may employ it. You may pick a mode, such as vibration, heat, air pressure, or music, according to your preferences. By your request, you may also modify the massage's duration and intensity.

You may prevent or relieve eye strain by using an eye massager in the afternoon, especially if you spend a lot of time in front of a computer, smartphone, or television. During your lunch break, or at other times you're feeling pressurized or weary, you may employ it for ten to fifteen minutes. You may pick a setting, such as heat, vibration, or music, to assist you rest your eyes. To power nap, you may also use an eye massager, which may help you fall asleep more quickly by shutting out light and noise.

In the evening, utilizing an eye massager may help you relax and get ready for a pleasant night's sleep, especially if you struggle to fall asleep or have insomnia. You may use it for ten to fifteen minutes during your TV or reading time, or before or after dinner. You may pick a setting, such as heat, music, or air pressure, that helps you relax. As melatonin, the hormone that governs your sleep cycle is created when you use an eye massager, you may also use it to increase the quality of your sleep.

How should I use an eye massager before, during, and after studying or working?

You may boost your attention and productivity before work or study by utilizing an eye massager, especially if you have a demanding or creative task ahead of you. You may use it for ten to fifteen minutes while planning or brainstorming, or before you begin working or studying. You may pick an air pressure, vibration, or music setting, for example, that stimulates your brain. An eye massager may also help you learn and recall things better as it stimulates the portions of your brain involved in these processes. When working or studying, employing an eye massager may help you remain focused and perform effectively, especially if you have a tiresome or long task ahead of you. You may use it whenever you're bored or distracted or for ten to fifteen minutes every hour or two. You may pick a mode—like heat, vibration, or music—that piques your senses. An eye massager may also help you feel less worried and nervous as it reduces the hormone cortisol, which is responsible for these symptoms. After work or study, employing an eye massager may help you relax and pamper yourself, especially if you've concluded a tough or gratifying task. You may utilize it for ten to fifteen minutes during your break from work or study, as well as for celebrations and contemplation. You may pick a setting, like music, heat, or air pressure, that settles your soul. Because an eye massager produces endorphins and serotonin, the chemicals responsible for these feelings, you may also use it to feel happier and more thankful.

How Can I Use an Eye Massager to Improve My Sleep, Relaxation, and Meditation?

You may better manage life's regular strains and tribulations by utilizing an eye massager as a form of relaxation, especially if you lead a busy or demanding lifestyle. If you need a break or a tranquil moment, or while you are involved in a pleasant or soothing activity, you may use it for ten to fifteen minutes. You may pick a mode (heat, vibration, air pressure, music) according to your mood. Because an eye massager may balance hormones and the nervous system, it may also balance the endocrine and neurological systems.

If your mind is racing or disorganized, employing an eye massager during your meditation sessions could help you acquire a degree of awareness and concentration. Whenever you desire to practice mindfulness or meditation, or if you're following a guided breathing exercise or meditation, you may employ it for ten to fifteen minutes. You may pick a mode—such as heat, music, or air pressure—that enhances your meditation. An eye massager may also help you open your crown and third eye chakras, which are energy centers that connect you to the divine and your higher self, which may help you meditate more profoundly and progress spiritually.

If you have a problematic or erratic sleep routine, utilizing an eye massager before bed could help you enjoy a more pleasant and refreshing sleep. Before going to bed or while lying in bed, you may use it for ten to fifteen minutes. You may pick a mode—like heat, air pressure, or music—that helps you fall asleep. An eye massager may also help you attain improved dream recall and lucid dreaming as it stimulates your pineal gland, which is responsible for creating DMT, the chemical that promotes these experiences.

How can I combine an eye massager with other treatments or products for eye care?

If you have a specific eye disease or concern, utilizing an eye massager in combination with other eye care products or treatments may help you maximize the benefits and effects of both. Depending on your preferences and your doctor's guidance, you may use an eye massager before, after, or in addition to other eye care products or treatments. You may pick a mode—such as air pressure, heat, vibration, or music—that works well with your eye care item or treatment. Because an eye massager may stimulate oxygen and blood flow to your eyes, you may also use it to promote the delivery and absorption of your eye care product or treatment.

You may use the following eye care goods or treatments in combination with an eye massager:

Eye drops

To distribute and retain the drops in your eyes, use an eye massager either before or after delivering the drops to lubricate and moisten them. To calm and relax your eyes, you may also use an eye massager in combination with eye drops.

Eye cream

To cleanse and exfoliate your eyes, use an eye massager before applying eye cream. To hydrate and nourish your eyes, use an eye massager after applying eye cream. To tighten and massage your eyes while you apply eye cream, you may also use an eye massager.

Eye mask

To prepare and open your eyes, use an eye massager before applying the mask. To close and refresh your eyes, apply an eye massager thereafter. To relax and massage your eyes, you may also use an eye massager in combination with an eye mask.

Eye surgery

You may use an eye massager to calm and relax your eyes before undergoing eye surgery, as well as to help your eyes heal and recover after it.

Moreover, you may support and massage your eyes with an eye massager while undergoing eye surgery.

How should you use an eye massager with your loved ones, friends, or partner?

If you have a close or personal connection, utilizing an eye massager with your spouse, family, or friends may help you have a delightful and peaceful experience. Depending on your schedule and preferences, you may employ both and one eye massager. You may pick a mode, like vibration, heat, air pressure, or music, that works best for your relationship. To strengthen your connection and communication, you may also apply an eye massager to promote empathy and trust.

Here are a few examples of ways to employ an eye massager with your loved ones, acquaintances, or partner:

With your partner

If your routine is boring or stressful, utilizing an eye massager jointly could bring some passion and compassion to your relationship. An eye massager may be used during or after intense kissing or cuddling. To express your love and dedication, you may also use an eye massager, which has the potential to create the hormone oxytocin, which is responsible for these feelings.

With your family

If your relationship with your family is tight or distant, utilizing an eye massager can allow you all to spend some quality time together and build your ties. During weekends, family get-togethers, and while playing video games or viewing movies, you may employ an eye massager. Since it may foster a sense of security and belonging, you may also use an eye massager to convey your support and care.

With your friends

If you lead a stressful or boring life, utilizing an eye massager with your friends may be a nice and soothing pastime. During get-togethers, sleepovers, parties, and talks, you may apply an eye massager. Because it may bring happiness and delight, you may also utilize an eye massager to commemorate your friendship and loyalty.

Chapter 3

Extra Hints and Techniques to Improve Your Eye Massager Experience

With the use of heat, vibration, and music, eye massagers are sophisticated devices that may help you relax, decrease eye strain, and increase your sleep. This chapter will cover how to personalize the settings and functions of your Eye Massager, how to use it with music, aromatherapy, or other sensory stimuli, how to use it to enhance your productivity, vision, and mood, how to use it to prevent or treat eye-related conditions or symptoms, and how to use it for enjoyment and fun.

How can I adjust the features and settings on my eye massager?

Your eye massager's model and brand will define which modification possibilities are available for its settings and functionalities. Among the common options and settings that you may alter are:

Temperature

Between 40°C and 42°C2, you may pick the optimum temperature for your eye massage. The heat may relieve eye strain, enhance blood flow, and relax the muscles surrounding your eyes.

Pressure

You select how vigorous the air pressure massage is; it varies from light to severe. The pressure can reduce headaches, calm anxiety, and stimulate the acupoints surrounding your eyes.

<u>Vibration</u>

You have the choice of picking an intermittent or continuous vibration massage frequency and mode. Your vision will be enhanced, your eyes will feel better, and you will be massaged by the vibration.

<u>Music</u>

During your eye massage, you may pick the sort and volume of music to play. It might be peaceful, stimulating, or relaxing. You may play your music playlists with your Eye Massager by linking it to your smartphone using Bluetooth. You may feel less stress, feel better, and relax with the music.

<u>Timer</u>

You get to pick how long to massage your eyes for—between 10 and 30 minutes. You can avoid overusing the timer by keeping note of how long you spend rubbing your eyes.

You may use the buttons on the machine, the remote control, or the accompanying smart app to adjust the settings and features of your eye massager. For subsequent use, you may also bookmark your favorite features and settings.

How can I employ Aromatherapy, music, or other sensory stimulation with an eye massager?

You may obtain even more benefits and a better eye massage experience by combining your eye massager with aromatherapy, music, or other sensory stimulants. The following are some recommendations for utilizing an eye massager in combination with aromatherapy, music, or other sensory stimuli:

Music

Listening to music may help you de-stress, feel happy, and relax. During your eye massage, you may pick the sort and volume of music that plays. It might be peaceful, energizing, or restful. You may play your music playlists with your Eye Massager by linking it to your smartphone using Bluetooth1. You may apply the following musical genres with your eye massager:

Classical music

You may boost your cognitive function, lower blood pressure, and relax your mind by listening to classical music.

Ambient music

This may assist in soothing the surroundings, decreasing anxiety, and facilitating sound sleep.

<u>Natural noises</u>

Natural sounds may enhance your immune system, increase your concentration, and make you feel more connected to the outdoors.

Binaural beats

These rhythms may help you relax, synchronize your brain waves, and increase your memory.

<u>Aromatherapy</u>

Aromatherapy helps balance your emotions, increase your well-being, and activate your sense of fragrance. When employing your eye massager, you may use candles, diffusers, sprays, or essential oils to create a pleasant smell in your home. You may use the following essential oils with your eye massager:

Lavender

Lavender contains relaxing, stress-relieving, and insomnia-easing effects.

Peppermint

Peppermint may assist with headache relief, vitality, and refreshment.

Rose

Rose may treat, relax, and raise your skin.

Chamomile

This plant contains relaxing, comforting, and anti-inflammatory qualities.

Additional sensory stimuli

You may create a multimodal experience by activating your senses beyond taste, touch, and proprioception with the assistance of extra sensory stimuli. To guarantee your comfort while using your eye massager, you may surround yourself with pillows, blankets, cushions, and other soft materials. While using your eye massager, you may also employ food, drinks, or supplements to refuel your body and mind. You may use the following as examples of meals, drinks, or supplements in combination with your eye massager:

Dark chocolate

This chocolate may increase your mood, sate your sweet yearning, and preserve your eyesight.

Green tea

This beverage may enhance your metabolism, help you detox, and keep you hydrated.

Omega-3

Omega-3 may aid in sustaining the health of your heart, brain, and eyes.

<u>Vitamin A</u>

This vitamin helps healthy skin, eyes, and immune systems.

How Can an Eye Massager Help You Be More Productive, Happy, and See Clearer?

Regular usage of your eye massager may boost your productivity, happiness, and vision. The following are some strategies for boosting your productivity, happiness, and vision by utilizing an eye massager:

Vision

By massaging your eyeballs, stimulating the acupoints surrounding your eyes, improving blood flow, and lowering eye strain, utilizing an eye massager may help you see better. You may strengthen your vision with your eye massager by:

★ Using it to decompress and prevent eye fatigue before or after working, studying, or reading.

★ Applying it to your eyes to correct and protect them from irritation, either before or after wearing glasses or contact lenses.

★ Applying it either before or after bed to moisturize and protect your eyes from dryness.

Mood

By relieving tension in your eyes, soothing your nerves, and playing music, utilizing an eye massager may raise your mood. You may enhance your mood with your eye massager by:

* Making use of it to alleviate stress and let go of emotions when you're feeling unhappy, worried, or pressured.

* Making use of it to excite your spirit and ignite your creativity when you're feeling depressed, uninspired, or bored.

* Making use of it to celebrate your successes and heighten your favorable feelings when you're feeling glad, appreciative, or satisfied.

Productivity

By boosting your vision, mood, and quality of sleep, utilizing an eye massager may help you be more productive. Your eye massager may help you be more productive in the following ways:

> ➤ Applying it first thing in the morning to awaken your eyes and give you a clear, bright view of the day.

> ➤ Applying it in the afternoon to boost energy, attentiveness, and eye refreshment.

> ➤ Applying it in the evening to relax and make your body and mind ready for a pleasant sleep.

How can I prevent or cure diseases or symptoms associated with my eyes using an eye massager?

By massaging your eyes with heat, pressure, and vibration, an eye massager may help you prevent or cure diseases or symptoms linked to the eyes. The following are some prevalent ailments or symptoms related to the eyes that an eye massager could help you prevent or relieve:

Eye strain

When your eyes are strained from heavy or prolonged use, such as reading, working, or driving, it is termed eye strain. Symptoms of eye strain include headaches, dry eyes, decreased vision, and eye pain. You may prevent or relieve eye strain by using your eye massager in the following ways:

→ Tailoring the vibration, pressure, and temperature settings to your comfort level and preferences.

→ Only use it for ten to fifteen minutes at a time, with intervals in between.

→ Using it to moisturize, strengthen, and calm your eyes in combination with eye exercises, eye drops, or eye patches.

Dark circles

A condition where the skin behind your eyes darkens more than the rest of your face, commonly as a consequence of allergies, age, genetics, or lack of sleep. Dark circles could create the appearance that you are older, sicker, or weary. You may prevent or get rid of dark circles by using your eye massager in the following ways:

★ **Raising the pressure and temperature settings to increase blood flow and minimize the look of pigmentation under your eyes.**

★ **Applying eye cream or serum after each session, and utilizing it for 15 to 20 minutes at a time.**

★ **Using it to protect, nourish, and rejuvenate your skin in addition to a balanced diet, appropriate sleep, and sun protection.**

Puffy eyes

This condition is brought on by swelling or inflammation of the skin around the eyes, which may be brought on by crying, allergies, fluid retention, or infections. You may look melancholy, unwell, or older than you are if you have puffy eyes. By utilizing your eye massager, you may decrease or prevent puffy eyes by:

☐ Lowering the pressure and temperature settings to decrease fluid accumulation and discomfort around your eyes.

☐ Use it for ten to fifteen minutes at a time. After each session, use your fingers to softly tap or massage your eyes.

☐ To calm, cool, and tighten your skin, use it in combination with tea bags, cucumber slices, or cold compresses.

CONCLUSION

We've learned how to enhance your Eye Massager experience with additional tips and methods in this chapter. We've talked about how to personalize your Eye Massager's settings and functions, how to use it with music, aromatherapy, or other sensory stimuli, how to use it to enhance your productivity, vision, and mood, how to use it to prevent or treat eye-related conditions or symptoms, and how to use it for enjoyment and fun.

With the use of heat, vibration, and music, the Eye Massager is a sophisticated device that may help you relax, reduce eye weariness, and increase your sleep. Through constant use of the Eye Massager and following the guidelines offered in this chapter, you may enjoy the benefits of the device and increase the health and general look of your eyes.

We hope that this book was enlightening and useful to you. Please give Eye Massager a try and let us know what you think.

www.ingramcontent.com/pod-product-compliance
Lightning Source LLC
Chambersburg PA
CBHW071000250726
48663CB00002B/309